Needing Cocaine

About the pamphlet:

Needing Cocaine is a collection of stories about people and their struggles with the powerful drug, cocaine. It shows the grip that drugs can have on individuals and their families, and describes the sometimes painful route back to sobriety. In *Needing Cocaine,* the anxiety, grief, anger, and denial of cocaine dependency is presented. But more important, the wonderful release from the power of drugs is shown, along with the healing effects of seeking help and working at a program for recovery. A brief history and pharmacology of cocaine is also included.

About the author:

Terry Webster is a free-lance writer who lives with his wife and daughter on a farm in rural, east-central Minnesota. In addition to working as a building contractor, he also finds time to do publicity writing for Hazelden and to work on ideas for future books.

Needing Cocaine

Terry Webster

Hazelden

First published May, 1985.

ISBN: 0-89486-260-X

Printed in the United States of America.

Editor's Note:

Hazelden Educational Materials offers a variety of information on chemical dependency and related areas. Our publications do not necessarily represent Hazelden or its programs, nor do they officially speak for any Twelve Step organization.

INTRODUCTION

Cocaine is a drug derived from the coca plant, which grows abundantly in the mountainous regions of South America. For centuries the natives of Peru, Columbia, Bolivia, and Ecuador have chewed raw coca leaves, enabling them to withstand, at least temporarily, the hardships of their daily lives. The use of coca is so widespread in these countries that a mouthful of leaves has come to represent a measure of walking time or distance. It has been estimated that up to 90% of the Andean Indian population chew coca leaves on a regular basis, and it is considered a necessity for long trips through the mountains.[1]

Chemists in Europe first isolated cocaine from the coca leaf in the middle 1800s, but it was used very little until the latter part of the century. An enterprising Italian, Angelo Mariani, concocted an elixer containing coca, which was sold throughout Europe in the late nineteenth century. Coca-Cola® was originally formulated from a combination of coca leaf and cola nut extracts. In 1904 the cocaine was removed from the popular drink and caffeine was used instead.

Sigmund Freud used the drug himself and experimented with cocaine on several of his patients as a treatment for alcoholism, morphine addiction, pain relief, and depression. He praised the drug for its apparently magical qualities and gave it to his relatives, colleagues, and fiancee. His dramatic description of cocaine's effects aroused great interest in the medical circles of the time. Freud stated that small doses of cocaine induced "exhilaration and lasting euphoria, which in no way differs from the normal euphoria of the healthy person. . . . You perceive an increase of self-control and possess more vitality and capacity for work. . . . In other words, you are simply normal, and it is soon hard to believe that you are under the influence of any drug. . . . Long intensive mental or physical work is performed without any fatigue. . . . This result is enjoyed without any of the unpleasant aftereffects that follow exhilaration brought about by alcohol. . . ."[2] Freud's enthusiasm for the drug diminished, however, as reports of severe addiction problems were published.

In 1914 the Harrison Narcotic Act mistakenly classified coca products as narcotics; since then the nonmedical sale, use, and possession has been illegal in this country. Cocaine smuggling into the United States was very limited until the 1960s, when increased law enforcement pressure on the amphetamine black market created a demand for a drug with similar effects. Since about 1980 cocaine has acquired an image identified with wealth, glamor, and beauty; it has become a symbol of success for many upwardly mobile members of the baby-boom generation. This image has also been attractive to many other people, regardless of their economic status; clinicians, social workers, and legal professionals are reporting a dramatic increase in problems associated with the use of cocaine.

Cocaine can be injected into muscles or veins, inhaled directly through the nose, or smoked in its freebase form. Eating the drug is relatively ineffective, because of slow absorption by the stomach and intestines.

Cocaine stimulates the central nervous system, producing effects similar to those of amphetamines. Physical effects include increased heart rate and blood pressure, numbing of mucus membranes, appetite suppression, and increased alertness and physical activity. The respiration rate initially rises sharply but then decreases. Conversely the body temperature drops at first, then rises above normal.

Users report euphoria, mental and physical stimulation, occasional mild hallucinations, and a pounding or throbbing in the ears. These sensations occur almost immediately and quickly build to a peak state referred to as a "rush" or "flash." Within a few minutes this subsides and is followed by intense feelings of confidence, omnipotence, and a state of high energy.

Regular cocaine users experience various side effects and aftereffects. Those who snort cocaine can have irritated sinuses, clogged, runny noses, and, occasionally, damaged nasal membranes. Intravenous users can suffer from collapsed veins or needle "tracks" from frequent injections, and other problems caused by unsanitary equipment or adulterants. Because the cocaine high is reached quickly and lasts a relatively short time, users often develop a pattern of repetitive and excessive use. Regardless of the method, frequent users can experience digestive disorders, nausea, loss of appetite, weight loss, insomnia, irritability, paranoia, and occasional violent behavior. Cocaine withdrawal causes chronic users to experience depression, anxiety, and a low emotional state (the "cocaine blues") which can lead to extreme paranoia and suicidal tendencies.

Although most research has failed to prove the existence of physical dependence, cocaine appears to be one of the most powerful psychological reinforcers known. One user, echoing a sentiment expressed by many, stated, "Once you try it, you want to try it again. If it is available to you, you keep on trying it until it becomes the passion of your life."

The following personal accounts are excerpts from interviews with people who have gone through the cocaine experience. Although the names, places, and details of their stories have been changed, the essence of their experience remains. They all have been in difficult situations, faced debilitating depressions, and endured losses that were hard for them to describe and sometimes hard to listen to. Yet, none of these people were extraordinary in their abilities to reshape their lives, or in their desire to overcome their addictions — except perhaps in one regard. Eventually they all accepted help and guidance when it was offered and made a commitment to themselves to do their best to live one day at a time.

The author is deeply grateful to these people for their time and willingness to share their personal stories so that others may listen and learn.

The author also wishes to thank the professional staff of Hazelden for their time, information, and support.

KATIE'S STORY

Katie walked briskly down the street, her purse swinging from her shoulder. It had been an exhausting, tense day at the office. Over the past eight hours she had typed boring letters, filed lifeless documents, and barked into the demanding phone. She was sure that four o'clock would never arrive, and when it did, she was out the door before anyone noticed. Although her job was more than three miles from home, Katie preferred to walk rather than wait for the unpredictable bus. She didn't look up as she passed the well-kept lawns littered with tricycles and trimmed shrubs. Katie was possessed with a single thought, and she needed to get home as soon as possible.

Jogging the last twenty steps on the hot asphalt driveway, Katie threw the heavy front door open and yelled with a voice that betrayed her edginess.

"I'm home! Jill, Chris, where are you?"

As she kicked off her shoes and hung her purse on the hook in the closet, she heard the low mumbling of the TV in the den. The kids had not heard her, or were more interested in the antics of the cartoon characters that glowed on the screen.

"John! Are you ready? I've had a hell of a day, I'm coming right up."

As Katie turned to climb the stairs she thought about checking in on the kids. They'll be OK for a few minutes, she thought, and besides, pretty soon I'll be in a better mood.

She thought of the ritual that was about to begin. Her husband, John, was probably getting the stuff out of the file box in the closet by now. Leaping two steps at a time, Katie reached the carpeted landing, grabbed the oak newel post, and pivoted her way around the left turn. She flew up the last four steps to the hallway, imagining the incredible contrast between how she felt now, and how she would feel in a short while.

"He'd better not be sleeping," she said silently; the thought made her angry.

"John? . . . where are you?"

"In here," came the reply from the bathroom off the master bedroom. "It's almost ready."

Katie stepped into the bathroom, turned quickly, and shut the door. She pushed in the brass button, locking out the rest of the world. The top of the toilet tank was leaning against the tub, and John was sitting backwards on the stool, hunched over the tank. He had a syringe in his hands, and as he drew water into it from the tank, he spoke slowly.

"Tough day, eh?"

"Yeah, the boss was mad because we lost a file somewhere, and the damn phone kept interrupting everything, and I ran out of speed at noon. I really am ready for this." Katie was repulsed by shooting up with water from the toilet tank. Even though John had reassured her many times that the water was just as clean as from the tap, she was still uneasy. But tonight she was willing to tolerate his little game, even though she knew he did it because it made her uncomfortable. Other than the source of the water, Katie loved the procedure of shooting coke. Her heart raced in anticipation as she plopped down on the floor, her back against the tub. She rolled up the left sleeve of her blouse and stretched out her arm.

John was now on his knees on the floor, using the toilet seat as a table. He measured out the fine, white powder into the spoon, added the water, stirred it gently with the needle tip, and drew the mixture into the syringe. When he had pulled up every drop, he pointed the needle at the gold plastic shower rod and snapped the side of the syringe with his finger. When all the air bubbles had risen to the tip, he turned to Katie, who had been watching him closely.

"Open up," he said, scooting over next to her. She opened her mouth and John squirted a thin stream of liquid mixed with air on her gums and tongue. Almost instantly her mouth started to numb. John held the syringe up to the light, checking for any potentially fatal bubbles. Finding none, he reached for a silk scarf and tied it tightly around her upper arm, looping the scarf so it could be released with a slight tug. Holding the needle in his left hand, John massaged Katie's arm on the inside of her elbow. He softly slapped the vein, trying to get it to swell and become more pronounced.

Katie had never injected herself; she had always been done by a man. Watching John prepare her fix, Katie felt real warmth for him. She saw his willingness to shoot her up as an expression of caretaking, and she knew this was the best kind of relationship she had experienced with a man. The bad parts of their marriage seemed to melt away when John injected drugs in Katie's veins.

Katie loved the ceremony, the intricate ritual that changed very little from one time to the next. But the preliminaries, which were both exciting and reassuring, were nothing compared to the incredible feeling that was about to happen.

John found the blood vessel with the needle point, and began easing in the plunger. Katie immediately closed her eyes, inclined her head to the side, and started to twitch slightly.

When she opened her eyes, she saw John leaning over her. He and the entire bathroom were shaking violently. She thought vaguely that he seemed to be shouting at her, but the pounding and throbbing in her ears were all she could hear. She was filled with pleasure from head to toe, and she closed her eyes to shut out the disturbing images. What a rush, she thought pleasantly.

"Katie, pull the scarf! Come on, you've got to loosen it!" demanded John. He had almost finished the injection, and it was time for Katie to untie the tourniquet. But she was not responding and her body was lurching uncontrollably. John quickly withdrew the needle and yanked the scarf free. He dotted an alcohol-soaked cotton ball on the needle site, then closed her forearm on it. The shaking subsided, but John could tell the dose was a little more than it should have been. He watched her for ten or fifteen seconds, trying to decide what to do, when suddenly her eyes popped open and her face broke out in a giant grin.

"Wow . . . that was *really* somethin'," she said. The words started coming quickly, and as she spoke, the tremor decreased to a small vibration. John knew she was OK, and as he listened to her stream on about the rush, her day at the office, and anything else that jumped into her head, he started to get his own fix ready. Downstairs, a small child whimpered at the sight of full-color, two-dimensional alien monsters, while his older sister told him to shut up.

> "I started using speed when I was thirteen years old. I got a prescription for diet pills, but I overused them. I only needed to lose about ten pounds, but I really enjoyed the feeling they gave me. I would tell my mother I lost them, and she would get the prescription refilled. This was in 1965, and diet pills were not considered speed; people didn't gasp when you mentioned them.
>
> "My parents were divorced when I was five years old, and my father died of alcoholism a few years ago. When I was thirteen my mother remarried; I hated my stepfather and stepbrother. I was very defiant, angry, and pretty much a loner. I wanted to lose weight because I thought it would help my social life. The pills made me feel self-confident and in control at a time when my life seemed uncontrollable.
>
> "I had one girlfriend in high school. We would drive to Iowa City and hang out on the university campus. We met older college kids, smoked pot, and drank alcohol. It made us feel like part of a group, and gave us a sense of belonging that was lacking at home. My school grades went down a little, but I had lost interest in school. I took easy classes and did just what was needed to get by. I spent all my time chasing my image of the world, longing to be part of it. And, increasingly, drugs became the

vehicle in which I imagined I could travel to that dream world."

After high school, Katie attended beautician's school. On weekends, she worked at a teenage nightclub, a place where kids gathered to dance and socialize. Katie got to know some of the band members, and soon learned that drugs were easily available. She would try anything, although she preferred the effects of amphetamines and other stimulants. Katie was starting to feel accepted by the group and comfortable with their lifestyle. She rebelled against anything that was not a part of this newfound sense of security. She isolated herself from her family and gradually lost interest in her career as a beautician. One day she had a woman with her head in the shampoo bowl, and Katie thought to herself, What do I need this for? I don't want to do it anymore. She packed her curlers in her bag and walked out, leaving the soapy-headed woman at the sink.

Katie continued to work at the nightclub and found another part-time job to help pay the bills. She was living away from home, had access to all the drugs she could afford, and had a circle of friends to share it with. During this time she took a lot of hallucinogens like LSD, psilocybin, mescaline, and peyote. She preferred speed, although she would smoke pot, drink booze, or take downers if nothing else was available. She loved the feeling of power and energy that uppers gave her.

There was something missing in Katie's life, but she wasn't sure what it was. One day in 1970, she headed west to the mountains. It was the continuation of a long journey in which drugs played an important role, and later the *most* important role.

During the next year, Katie moved around a lot, living with different people, working various jobs, even attending college for one quarter. She also helped start a locally successful underground newspaper. It was at this time that Katie met Hank, a wanderer from Oklahoma. Hank had no job, received money from his folks, and mainlined speed and cocaine whenever he could get it. He and Katie got an apartment together, and between his money from home, and her job as a secretary, they managed to keep themselves in food and drugs. Although Katie watched Hank shoot up many times, she only took drugs orally. She felt that by not mainlining, she didn't have a problem. Eventually though, Hank's descriptions of the rush and excitement convinced her to give it a try.

"I loved it. There is nothing in the world like shooting coke. I never wanted to do drugs in any other way again. It was a completely physical thing for me, from top to bottom — every inch of my body. It took no time at all for it to happen, for that good, 'filled-up' feeling to start. Sometimes, when he was in a hurry he would want to snort it, and I would get upset. I would say, 'What a waste, why not spend the extra time and do it right?'

"After Hank and I split up, I met my husband, John. We lived together for a while; then we got married. We spent almost all of our time together doing drugs. Those years are real foggy to me. I don't remember a lot of details. We had two kids, Jill and Chris. I stopped taking drugs when I was pregnant, but started again after they were born. Those were real crazy years.

"Sometimes we would go into the mountains for the weekend, and bring along a few hundred dollars worth of coke. We'd put the kids to bed in the tent, and start shooting coke — all night long. One time we ran out on a Saturday afternoon; we loaded up the kids and everything and headed back to town where we could score more coke.

"We bought a $100,000 house in Colorado Springs. I was working as a secretary, bringing home $350 a week, and John worked as a subcontractor. We probably could have managed if it weren't for the money we spent on drugs. I don't remember a time when we didn't use all the drugs we had. Then we would try and buy some more;

even if the mortgage was due, we would take whatever cash we had, and buy what we could get. About this time we figured out that by dealing we could get our stuff cheaper. We even thought we could get rich by dealing! We were sure wrong."

"Get a sitter for tonight, OK? We're going over to Manuel and Jody's place — they got some fine stuff, and Frank wants us to score for him." John had business on his mind, and he expected Katie to make the arrangements for the kids if she wanted to join him.

"Yeah, sure. Did Frank sell another house? How much does he want this time?" Katie knew that when their realtor friend closed on a house deal it meant lots of money for coke, which meant lots of coke for John and Katie.

"He gave me $5,000 this afternoon."

On the way over in the car, John told Katie not to ask any questions at Manuel and Jody's. He didn't have to remind her; she didn't want to know very much about dealing anyway. As he neared the house, John looked up and down the street, checking for anything suspicious. He drove past their place, and parked in front of a house halfway down the block. As Katie stepped out onto the sidewalk, she clutched her purse in her left hand while slamming the rusty door of the Ford. John walked around to the back of the car, and taking a quick glance at the neighborhood, opened the trunk. He reached inside and grabbed an old green army backpack, jerked the key from the lock, and slowly closed the trunk. He was careful not to let it latch, so that it could be opened quickly without the key.

Katie and John walked casually down the sidewalk toward Manuel and Jody's. They said nothing to each other, trying to appear calm and cool on the outside. Inside John's dusty backpack was $5000 in cash.

"Stand next to me, so he can see your face," said John as he knocked on the door. There was an anxious moment while the occupants presumably looked over the visitors. Then the door

door pulled quickly open, while John and Katie stepped into the foyer. Just as quickly the door was closed behind them.

"John, good to see ya, man. Howja make out with your friend, the house pusher?"

"I got it right here, in the bag. Five big ones." John smiled as they walked into the living room. There were seven or eight people laying around on the floor and furniture. It was obvious that the party had already started.

As Katie plopped down on the couch, she noticed the coffee table in front of her. Scattered in among the chips, cheese, and bottles of wine were piles of money. She could see lots of fifties and hundreds, and several five hundred dollar bills.

"Wow, like, how much is there?" she asked Jody who was sitting next to her.

"With the fiver that you guys brought, that should make . . . oh, about a half-million."

Katie was stunned. This was more than she had ever seen, or thought about. She was suddenly very paranoid.

John had been over in the corner of the room, hunched over a small table with Manuel. He came over and sat on the floor next to Katie, opened the backpack, which he had not let go of since they came, and showed her the contents. Inside, white and shiny from the plastic coverings, were several tightly rolled bags of cocaine. As Katie pulled a syringe from the stash bag, John carefully opened one of the baggies. Someone put a Creedence Clearwater record on the turntable, while Manuel stood on a chair, making a speech. As her rush subsided, Katie heard Manuel say, "So, what we need is someone to drive this cash to Miami, see, and then you just park it there and get on a plane and fly back. Nothing to it. And, of course, whoever does it will get a nice cut of the action. . . ."

> "Initially, we were real honest when we were dealing. We just sold to close friends, we were just middlemen. But eventually we'd take the stuff home and try a little bit for ourselves. All of a sudden it would be two days later

and we had shot up $1,000 worth of someone else's cocaine. So we'd cut it with whatever we could find. Sometimes we'd say we couldn't get any, and when people would want their money back we'd go to the bank and remortgage the house. We did that three or four times, and finally the bank started to foreclose. We always thought that we could get it back by making a big buy and selling it all, but we would always end up shooting up the profits, and then some. Somehow I was able to keep my job, even though I'd usually go to work 'flying.' All my money would go for paying off drug debts, and I'd buy food and clothes for the kids on my credit cards.

"Finally we couldn't do it anymore. Everything fell apart. Our marriage ended in divorce. Since we had both been doing drugs since we were kids, our emotional development was stopped at about the age of fourteen. When we weren't high, we were fighting. I knew when he was on the verge of hitting me, and the closer he got, the more I'd taunt him. He hit me with a lamp once, and beat my head against a wall. I became very suspicious and hateful. The members of his family were enablers, but they were loving and they cared. I would get coked-up and write them horrible letters telling them how terrible they were. Everything became very, very ugly.

"Toward the end of my drug use, coming down was terrible. I would get a headache shortly after the initial rush. The only thing that made it go away was to shoot more coke. In a little while, the headache would start to come back. So I'd do more coke, and keep up the pattern until there was none left. As I did the last bit, I would think about coming down, anticipating what it was going to be like, how awful it was. If I had some downers I'd take those, and sleep it off. But if there was nothing, I'd suffer. I hated the suffering. Coming down was a real panic, very desperate. I would think, my God, my world is ending.

"Everything became urgent; I felt I needed to do something right away, but I had no idea what to do. I would keep busy and behave as if I were still flying, but I would get scattered and do half of twenty different things. I'd cry, start fights with my husband, and blame him because we were out of coke. I would yell at the kids, and get into irrational arguments with people over things that didn't matter. I can remember licking the mirror, putting water in the needle and shooting it in my mouth, hoping that there was something there that could make it not feel so bad. Eventually I would just lie down and pray that I could go to sleep. It would feel like eternity, but I suppose it was only six or eight hours.

"It was like that all the time the last few months I was using. The highs never lasted, the lows were at rock-bottom, and life was impossible to live. I never tried to kill myself, but I thought about it sometimes."

Katie had spent many years learning her denial system. She told herself she had no problem with drugs, because she didn't fit her image of a drug addict. In the early years, taking speed was OK, because "They were only diet pills, and a doctor prescribed them." Later, she justified her consumption of various pills by assuring herself that she wasn't using needles, so she couldn't have a problem. Then, when she started mainlining amphetamines and cocaine, she knew she was all right because, as she told herself, "I don't shoot heroin — I'm no junkie." This self-deception ultimately caught up with her. She was exhausted — physically, emotionally, and financially. Katie was lucky, in one sense. One day all the pieces came together, and she saw that she was in trouble, and needed help.

Katie continued going to work and somehow managed to make it through most days. Her fellow workers thought her eccentric, but few suspected the trauma she was living. During the day she typed letters, but at night she went to bars, looking for men to buy her drinks or give her drugs. Some mornings it took a lot of "white crosses" to get it together enough to continue.

One morning she was awakened by her aunt who had come by to care for the children while Katie went to work. Her aunt asked her what had happened to her face, and when Katie got up and looked in the mirror, she was shocked. There were bruises all over her head and neck, scrapes and scratches, and dried blood. And the injuries were not limited to her head; she was covered from top to bottom with gashes and black-and-blue marks. Katie weakly stared in the mirror, and sat down hard on the bed. She assumed that she had been beaten up, but she had no recollection of what had happened. Try as she might, she could remember nothing past meeting some guys in a bar and having a few drinks.

Finally, Katie was scared. This missing part of her life, with such dramatic results, frightened her a great deal. She reached for the phone. Her ex-husband, John, had gone through treatment a few months before, and she knew a friend who attended Al-Anon. They both told her that she needed to call Alcoholics Anonymous, and when she did, she talked to a woman who listened to her. Katie was lonely, scared, and she could not continue living the way she was. But after sixty days she had formed the basis for a new, healthy, drug-free life.

> "I'm going to complete the program I'm in now. I have the ability to finish it, and it will be the first real thing that I've completed since high school. It's real hard. I've got the kids, and finances are real tight, but the money comes. I worry about it sometimes, but it will happen somehow. It has to. I am going to make it.
>
> "I never see the people I did drugs with; the minute I quit, they disappeared. But the people I've met in A.A. are wonderful. I've known them a short while, and they come and visit the kids and me. They really care about what happens to me. I never experienced that before — the encouragement, the caring, the positive feelings.

"John and I are going to try a reconciliation. We always loved each other, but there was so much sickness in our lives that we couldn't find the good things. It won't be easy. Our lives have changed so much since we stopped using drugs that we feel we hardly know each other. But we both think it's worth a try.

"I thought I was using drugs, but they were really using me. I never got what I wanted out of drugs. How do you make people believe they are going to die unless they quit using? *I* didn't believe it. I didn't need to destroy my liver, have high blood pressure, go through the D.T.s, or rupture a vein. I could have died because I couldn't see straight to drive; because I got in with people who didn't care about me.

"There were a lot of years that I could have done something with. I'm starting where most people are when they're twenty — trying to make a career, deciding what to do with my life, making enough money to survive. I'll be paying that mortgage for years. I can't get credit cards because I was over $7000 in debt to Visa and Mastercharge. That's OK, because I got a second chance, but I wonder how many chances there are out there. I don't want to find out.

"Coke will eat you alive. People consider cocaine to be glamorous, attractive. What can be glamorous about sitting on a bathroom floor with a rag tied around your arm, shaking, waiting for someone to stick a needle in you? Cocaine is a very powerful drug and it's not classy, not at all. Of all the drugs that I did, I think I feel OK about never again taking most of them. But I have a sense of loss for cocaine. I thought it filled up all the empty places. But I am very grateful to be done with it. The only real freedom is to do what you should do, because you want to. And I really want to, and I will."

DANA'S STORY

Dana grew up on a family farm in western Minnesota. He had six brothers and sisters, and they all had to work hard to make the operation successful. His memories are of feeding hogs, milking cows, baling hay, and many hours of driving a tractor. There wasn't a lot of time for anything not directly related to farming, except school, and even that was restricted to the regular school day. Dana participated in few extra-curricular activities while in school. He seemed to have little interest in sports, art, drama, or other school clubs. He was socially isolated from most of his peers, partly because of his home responsibilities, and partly because of his quiet nature.

After high school, Dana went to a small, private college in a large city, where he lived alone in an off-campus apartment. At first he worked hard and kept his grades up. However, he was very lonely. He knew a few people from his classes, but he rarely saw them outside of the classrooms. Midway through the second quarter, Dana's feelings of loneliness overtook his sense of insecurity, and he started going to bars on the weekends. There, with the aid of alcohol, he made friends.

"Liz, I'd like you to meet a friend of mine. Dana, this is Liz. Dana is in his second quarter and majoring in plants or something. Liz is studying Roman stuff. I'm gonna go pick up Sally, so you two get acquainted and we'll see you in a bit."

Steve breezed out of the smoky bar, leaving Dana nervous. Thank heavens he had drunk a few beers before meeting his blind date. But another one might help calm him down.

"Would you care for a beer?" he asked, with all the false bravado he could muster.

"Oh, sure," Liz replied.

As Dana made his way through the crowded room to the bar, he thought about making a break for the door. It had nothing to do with Liz, it was just his shyness and lack of self-confidence. But he decided against it and returned with a pitcher of beer.

"So, old Romans, huh? History or art?" Dana hated small talk. It seemed so artificial and it made him nervous.

"History, I guess," said Liz. "Pretty boring stuff, actually. You know, poets and philosophers and government types. I'm gonna switch to a different major next quarter. I think maybe I'd like to go into broadcasting — being a TV anchor woman might be neat. So, what do you do with plants?"

As they talked, Dana noticed his palms were still sweating. The beers had undoubtedly helped, but he wished that Steve would hurry back. He filled his mug from the pitcher, and reached across the table to top off Liz's glass. As he tried to describe his educational plans, Dana slipped and poured cold beer over the side of her glass and onto the table.

"Say, listen. You seem a little uptight," said Liz as she wiped the beer with a napkin. "Wanna smoke a joint?"

Dana had never taken any drugs, other than alcohol, but if it would calm his nerves it might be worth a try.

"Ah . . . sure, I guess. Only I'm a little out of practice with that stuff."

As they made their way to the parking lot they ran into Steve and Sally. The four of them hopped into Steve's car and drove out into the countryside.

Before long, Dana was trying all kinds of drugs, from marijuana to LSD to speed, and enjoying the feelings that they gave him. By the end of the third quarter, Dana was smoking pot and taking "white crosses" almost every day. He still managed to keep up with most of his schoolwork, but he was starting to care less and less.

During this period, a typical day for Dana would begin with his alarm going off at 10:00 A.M. If he got up right away, he could make it to his first class at 10:30. But usually he was nursing a hangover, so he would lay in bed a while, trying to decide if there was any compelling reason to go to class. By 10:15 he would be rummaging in his dresser drawer looking for socks and his stash of drugs. Depending on his mood, he might decide to smoke a joint on the way to class, or maybe take a few hits of speed. Regardless, he would stumble into his biochemistry lab or plant propagation lecture high as a kite, and usually late. His professors occasionally scolded him, but they could tell by his grades that school was not very important to him.

Dana's parents were financing his education, and they sent him money every month. They made sure that he had enough for the basics — food, rent, tuition, and books — plus they always sent extra "pocket money," which he used to buy drugs. It wasn't long before he would run out of drugs before his next check from home would arrive. At this point, his friend Steve talked him into doing a little dealing.

"So, ya see, if you have enough cash to buy the thousand hits of zip, then you can sell 900 or so, and have the rest free. Same thing with the pot. Buy a pound, and get a lid for yourself. All you need is cash up-front, and you can turn it over as fast as you want.

While Steve talked, Dana was listening to him with one ear, hearing the bar band with his other ear, and trying to make sense out of all of it. He and Steve had smoked a couple of joints before they got to the bar, where they had downed two pitchers of beer.

"How much would I need?" asked Dana, not sure that he could come up with very much cash.

"Oh, four, maybe five hundred would get a good start. After you've been doing it a while, you might get the supplier to front you the stuff ahead of time. Then you're in the clear."

Suddenly Dana figured it out. His folks sent him $600 a

month for his expenses. They always sent the money a couple of weeks in advance. If he could only turn the stuff around in two weeks, he would be in business.

Dana became the center of attention in his new-found circle of friends. He was the guy who could get just about any drug, even on short notice. He imagined himself making big money, as well as having many friends. But even though people were always calling him and he was selling quite a bit, it wasn't working out. He found that he still had a deep feeling of emptiness inside that his "friends" were not filling up. When he took drugs he could forget that empty feeling for a while. With his increasing usage, however, he found that he wasn't making the big money he had expected. Dana was able to purchase a bag of speed, or a pound of pot, repackage it in small quantities, sell it for what he had paid, and have enough drugs left over to keep him going for a while. At least, he thought, I figured it out so it's not costing me anything to use.

After spring break, his supplier turned him on to cocaine for the first time. The experience was a real milestone in Dana's career as a drug dealer. Cocaine became very important to him, and he loved the power and self-satisfaction that it gave him. Although he was unable or unwilling to see it, Dana's life was well on the way to becoming an unmanageable mess.

> "That first time, I thought it would be really great to snort some good coke. I had heard all about it, how wonderful it made you feel, how it wasn't addictive, how it was a high-class drug. I found that I really enjoyed cocaine, that it made me feel warm inside. I really got off on the whole thing — not just the high, but the taste, the ritual. I savored the process of chopping it with a razor blade, lining it up on the mirror, licking the razor, snorting it through a rolled up $20 bill, then the incredible rush, the feeling of numbness, and going around sniffling afterwards. I especially liked it when I combined it with

other drugs. I loved snorting and drinking, they just seemed to go together for me.

"Since I always enjoyed the prestige of being able to sell high-quality drugs, I was sure that I would make a lot of money by dealing coke. I figured if I bought six grams, sold five and a half and snorted a half gram myself, I would be able to make $100 cash. Unfortunately, few people at school could afford much coke, and it didn't sell very fast. So I had it sitting around, in my drawers or closets, just begging to be used. I thought if I snorted just one more line, it would only be a *little* less profit. What usually happened was I sold two or three grams, and snorted three or four, and lost money. And if I lost a little this month, I could always make it up next month. I always believed that since I *had* to make the money back, I would.

"Sometimes, when I'd buy a quarter ounce, I'd bag it all up and get it ready to sell. After a week or so I'd use up the stuff I had set aside for myself and still have four or five grams left to deal. So I'd go through each bag and take a little bit out so I could get high. It didn't bother me that I was shorting my friends. If it still hadn't all sold by the time I had snorted that, I would just take one of the remaining bags, and make it mine.

"So one month I didn't have enough money to pay my tuition. I had snorted up all my profits, and justified it to myself by thinking I'd do better next time. I had to borrow money from friends to buy food and pay the rent. I made up some excuse to the school admissions office, and they let me continue taking classes without full payment.

"Every month the unpaid tuition bill became higher, and I owed money to friends and for bills. As the sum increased, my rationalization for snorting became, 'Well, when I get a summer job, it will only take one day to pay for this line.' I felt that I could toot without feeling guilty since I was willing to pay for it all — some day. And besides, the coke and other drugs made it real easy to forget all my problems."

During this period Dana became increasingly depressed and unhappy. He became more and more uncomfortable around people, and would often lock his door and pretend he wasn't home. He was using a wide variety of drugs, and would self-prescribe his chemicals, based on what his mood was like. Dana enjoyed the effects of acid and he would take a hit of that, and a few hours later smoke some pot to calm down. Then he would take speed or coke to cheer up, and to make him feel like going to class.

On one occasion, Dana spent four days locked in his room with the lights out and shades drawn, snorting coke and drinking vodka. He ignored the telephone and refused to answer the door. Later, after the binge was over, he gruffly told friends that he had "been away for a few days."

Dana's grades had fallen, and he often skipped classes. When he did show up, he was usually high on something, and would sit alone in a corner. He avoided social contact with everyone, except his drug supplier and a few of his drug customers. Eventually he became an almost total recluse. The lifestyle that was exciting and social had become depressing, antisocial, and desperate. Dana had withdrawn into a world inside his own mind.

Dana's sister, Mary, was familiar with a chemical dependency treatment center near her home. She knew he was having trouble at school, with his finances, and with their parents. Mary guessed that drugs were a big part of Dana's life, and she tried to convince him to get help. At first he refused, stating that he had no problems, but he accepted her invitation to visit her for a few days. During the course of the visit, Mary listened to Dana describe his life, and she told him what she knew about drug usage. She tried to get him to participate in an assessment interview at the treatment center, but his denial was still too great. He returned to school, and Mary worried about what would happen to him.

Dana had decided to prove to Mary, and to himself, that he could easily control his drug use. He intended to stay clean for at least a week. That would prove that he was still in charge, and that he had no problems with drugs.

Dana spent the first day back from his sister's house cleaning his apartment. He skipped his classes because he wanted to avoid all of his friends. As he scrubbed the bathtub and washed the stacks of dirty dishes he thought to himself that going straight was going to be a snap. That evening, after zealously putting his apartment back together, he went to bed early. Although he had a rather fitfull night's sleep, interrupted by several bad dreams, the next morning Dana felt rested and ready to attend school. He arrived on time for his first class, sat near the front of the room, and took copious notes on the lecture. About halfway through the class Dana became aware of a slight headache. But in his fervor to succeed at school and with his "experiment," he ignored the uncomfortable sensation.

As the day wore on, the headache became more intense, and Dana's mood changed from optimistic self-pride to agitated nervousness. By the end of the day he was distraught and uncomfortable. He went home, popped the top on a beer "to take the edge off," and tried to study. After three beers and a shot of vodka, Dana got out his bag of coke and snorted a long line. He didn't think about his previous vow to abstain from drugs for a week. All he thought about was the pleasure that was running through him; he tossed his books under the couch and turned on the television. Dana was off on a big binge.

A few days later Mary got a phone call from Dana. He had been high for three days, and had used up his drugs. He knew that he wasn't able to control his drug usage and was willing to try the treatment center.

> "Mary was always willing to listen and talk with me, and she was the one person I was not afraid to talk to. When I got sick enough, I went to the assessment interview. While I was there, I realized that I was powerless

over drugs, and I decided to go into treatment. It was difficult, and I had to face up to a lot of things I had tried to bury with drugs. After treatment, I went to A.A. meetings and sometimes I was extremely depressed and uncomfortable. One month after completing treatment, I went out and got high. I went on a two-day binge, but when I sobered up I called my A.A. sponsor. I eventually lived in a halfway house for a while, and today I am very grateful that I have been clean for over three years. I go to both A.A. and Narcotics Anonymous meetings regularly.

"One day during treatment, with the prodding of a friend, I came to realize I couldn't make myself better alone — I needed help with that. That was very important for me; afterwards, I just kept coming back to those meetings. Much of my old sickness has gradually subsided, and my real personality has appeared to fill up the space left by the drugs. Since I really don't want to go back to my old life, I'm willing to work at the program, even though it is sometimes very hard. But there are a few things that I know for sure now: there are people around me who understand, care, and sincerely want to help me; I don't have to fight with drugs constantly; and I enjoy being alive, which is not how it used to be.

"Before I found out there was help available, I felt completely alone and hopeless. It was hard for me to see that that could change, but it did. Now I know a lot of people just like me, and that is a very good feeling."

ALAN'S STORY

Hernandez smiled as he looked into the full-length mirror. He had never dreamed he would be dressed in such exquisite fashions, or be part of the fast society world of Boston. He had come a long way from the slums of Buenaventura, Columbia. Alan had taken his friend Hernandez to one of the most exclusive men's clothiers in Boston, and was outfitting him in the latest European style — three piece suit, silk tie, wing tips, the works.

Alan and Hernandez left the shop with packages in their hands and hangers draped over their shoulders. The humid air made the thin plastic clothing bags stick to their necks. It was a short distance to where their Jaguar was parked and as they sped off down the street they discussed the plans for the evening — or rather, Alan discussed them. Hernandez spoke and understood only basic English, and Alan's rapid fire conversations often left him confused. Alan aimed the car towards the wealthy suburb where they lived, while the wipers slapped steadily at the raindrops.

"So, we're going to the Redfern Athletic Club tonight! Listen, we'll pick up Amy and Sue at seven o'clock and then we'll head out to the club for dinner and maybe a little tour. Then, a little later on. . . ."

Alan chattered on about the evening arrangements, stopping every few minutes to let Hernandez hold a small spoon under his right nostril. Alan sniffed the fine white powder deeply into his nose, and Hernandez reached over and operated the steering wheel. Somehow they made it home, got themselves dressed, and drove to the street corner where the women were waiting for them.

"Good evening Mr. Turner. May I show you to your table?" The maitre d' slipped through the crowded dining room, escorting the recent Columbian immigrant, the wealthy businessman, and their two prostitutes to Alan's private table. Everyone ordered drinks and Alan passed a small packet across the table to one of the women.

"Here's a partial payment," he said with a laugh. "Let's have some fun tonight!"

The women smiled and left for the restroom, taking the packet along. When they returned, Alan was ordering dinner for everyone. It didn't occur to him to ask the others what they preferred. This was his show and he would put it on any way he wanted.

> "I have always been a good businessman, and I knew that at a hundred dollars a gram, cocaine was a rip-off. I figured it could be gotten at a lower price and higher quality. So, I started getting to know the people I was buying from, ingratiating myself, and gradually working my way up to their supplier. There were five levels between the people who were selling grams and this Columbian named Hernandez. The others were taking care of him, but he spoke little English, and they were ripping him off. I eventually got to know him, took him out and bought him clothes, rented an apartment for him, and arranged for prostitutes to visit him. I had completely locked up my source of supply and became a partner with Hernandez. He had all the contacts for purchasing the coke, and I had the money to front him and the sources to sell it to."

"Waiter . . . waiter!" Alan snapped his fingers impatiently, raising his voice so that other patrons of the club's dining room turned to stare. "Get me the manager!" he demanded.

As soon as the waiter had rushed off, Alan, Hernandez, and the two women started to giggle uncontrollably. They had made repeated trips to the rest rooms, and the cocaine combined with the champagne had made them rather giddy. As the manager of the club walked toward them, however, Alan hissed at them to "straighten up and fly right!"

"Yes, Mr. Turner, what can I do for you?" asked the very proper manager. He had known Alan for many years, and had experienced his strange behavior on several occasions. He half-expected to be insulted or threatened.

"Mr. Schneider, may I present Hernandez Guacamole. He is a close family friend and is in town doing some work for his father. Mr. Guacamole is a very wealthy manufacturer from Columbia and is considering building some warehouses here in Boston. We were wondering if we might arrange to have a tour of the facilities this evening. Hernandez's family is very large and I would think if the club meets their standards, several of them would be interested in becoming members."

The manager hesitated, then smiled broadly while pumping Hernandez's hand. "I would be pleased to show you the club myself! Send for me after your meal." As the manager walked away he caught the waiter's attention and had him deliver a bottle of French wine to the table, gratis.

"The whole story was totally made up, right down to the absurd last name. We had a great time that night, pulling that manager's leg. He fell all over Hernandez, tried everything to impress him, to entice him to become a member. And, of course, Hernandez understood very little of what was going on — he just knew he was having the best time of his life.

"As we were escorted around the club we entered practically every rest room, and once inside would burst out laughing. While the manager waited patiently in the corridor, we snorted long lines of cocaine off of the sink tops. Eventually, he showed us the private rooms that could be rented. They were like exclusive hotel rooms, with saunas and whirlpools. We rented one for the night, had several bottles of wine and scotch sent up, and enjoyed the company of our female companions until the wee hours. It was incredibly outrageous, and very expensive — but neither money nor morals mattered to me at that time.

"I saw my life as full and vibrant, exciting and adventurous. But I still hadn't faced one important fact: I didn't have everything I needed, and I was trying to fill that void with drugs.

"I grew up in an emotionally isolated family. I knew my parents loved me, but there was no touching or hugging, no closeness or displays of affection. Sex was never discussed, feelings were not shared — it was not considered 'good form.'

"I was an only child and grew up in a very controlled environment. I didn't do many of the things 'normal' kids did. I had a daily schedule of studying at home, even during the summer. I knew I would take over the family insurance business and there was a lot of pressure to do well. I remember crying when I was in sixth grade because I had received low grades. I was afraid I wouldn't be accepted to the college my father attended. One year I really wanted to go to summer camp in the mountains. A month in the wilds — swimming, hiking, being normal. Instead, I had to stay home and take golf lessons. I was very angry, but I soon buried that anger, with all my other emotions.

"I was accepted at my father's college and did fairly well in school. But I learned I could drink more than most other people. I'd be drunk from Friday evening to Sunday afternoon, when I would go to the library and start studying again. I got used to that binge syndrome of being able to work hard when I had to, and play hard when the work was done.

"After college, my father's business took a lot of effort. My drinking tapered off, but I was not very happy. I would blame my wife for my dissatisfactions with myself and with the business. Eventually, I started drinking more on weekends with the cocktail crowd. After ten years of this behavior, I decided I could start drinking Friday evening, and then Friday noon. On weekends, when there were large parties to attend, I would get very drunk; my behavior became quite obnoxious.

"One occasion showed me how far I had gone. I got very drunk at a formal dinner and made a pass at the elderly wife of one of the other guests. When I woke up the next day, I was mortified, shocked that I could be so disgusting. I never wanted to drink again.

"I told a neighbor I wanted to quit drinking, but was having trouble stopping. He took me to an Alcoholics Anonymous meeting and I attended meetings for about two years, but the group didn't focus on A.A.'s Twelve Steps as much as I needed. I wasn't working any kind of program, and was still unhappy. I stopped attending the meetings, and stayed sober for about four years. But though I wasn't drinking, I was still quite obnoxious and belligerent, and this caused a lot of problems with my wife and others.

"After spending fourteen years in my father's insurance business, I was burned out. I was still trying to please my father, even though I really wanted to do something different. I had tripled the company's size, yet he could only criticize me for having too many expenses. I think this may have been part of my just giving up.

"At about this time, several things happened that allowed me to give up my sobriety and continue even further towards self-destruction."

"Hilary, do you remember Mr. Gibson from Gibson International Services? He called and would like to treat us to a vacation in Ireland for a week. I told him that we'd be delighted." Alan enjoyed springing surprises on his wife, and he hoped this one would help mend their relationship. Lately they had been seeing less of each other, and their time together was full of tension.

"When is it, Alan?" Hilary wondered if she could tolerate an entire week with Alan. It wasn't that she didn't love him, it was just that he wasn't very pleasant to be around. He was hot-tempered, gruff, and angry much of the time.

"We'll leave this Friday."

"Alan, you know that Dave and Sandy are coming this week-end. I haven't seen them in six years! I cannot just go flitting off to Ireland and cancel the plans I've made with them!" Hilary was amazed at his gall. He really expected her to go along with him.

"Well, then I'll just find someone else who is interested in experiencing a different culture. For free, no less!"

Alan called a friend and the two of them made the flight across the ocean. In Ireland, Alan decided that he should really try some of the native stout ales. He hadn't had any alcohol for almost four years, but he didn't seem to have any problem the first night. The second night he had a dozen ales, and he drank away the rest of the trip.

After his return to Boston, his drinking started to increase dramatically, and he started experimenting with other drugs, mostly marijuana.

A few months later, Alan's mother died. His father asked him whether he was planning on wearing his blue pinstripe suit or his plain blue suit to the funeral. That was the extent of their conversation about his mother's death. After the funeral they had a catered reception at the house, went to the country club for dinner, and went to work the next day. Grieving was not "good form" either.

> "I started drinking very heavily after my mother's death. I got into more trouble with my wife, became even more obnoxious, and she moved to a small apartment and left me with this huge house. So I sat around all by myself and I started feeling very lonely.
>
> "I started going to singles bars because I needed companionship, and I didn't know where to find it. I tried

some cocaine and didn't even get high the first time, but I found that a lot of women were interested in doing coke. It was always very scary for me to ask a woman out for a drink, but to ask them if they wanted to do some coke was emotionally much safer.

"Things started at the gram level, which would last me a few weeks. I had no problems at all with the drug. This went on for a few months. Then I met Hernandez, and I figured out I could get the cost down by going in with him. At this point I was using two to three hundred dollars worth on the weekends.

"Soon my use progressed from a couple grams a week to a gram every evening. I'd go to singles bars every night and drink, snort coke, and pick up women. I was staying out later and later. Soon I closed the bars every night, and often went home and continued using drugs.

"I was able to run the insurance business almost entirely from my house. I would call my biggest clients, but everything else I could delegate. I think my employees were afraid to confront me, but I paid everybody well enough so they covered for me. By that point I was just keeping things going so that I could have the money to buy drugs and sex.

"My cocaine use climbed to at least a gram and a half every day, and I started keeping it in my office and cars. I'd toot a few lines before going on business calls. I'll bet I made some pretty interesting impressions on a few people.

"After a year of using cocaine, I was completely out of control. I had wild parties with other addicts, prostitutes, and underworld figures who carried guns. I became obsessive in my possesion of drugs, and my behavior had become increasingly bizarre. I wanted to try any kind of deviant behavior I could imagine. I engaged in a lot of crazy sexual acting-out. I got into using a lot of hookers. I would have one show up at the house at seven o'clock, then she would leave at eight and another would arrive. Then another would come at ten and stay until midnight. I had a three page notebook full of women's names and phone numbers. Sometimes, if they had other clients who wanted to act something out with a man, I would go along.

"I was always shy and insecure, but I had a lot of money, and I found when I had a big bag of cocaine I became very popular. It was a powerful feeling to be able to pull out an ounce of cocaine — most people only saw grams. I could attract a lot of women who wanted to get high. Part of it was sex, but part of it was so I could control them, have power over them, manipulate them.

"I started a sexual relationship with a fourteen-year-old girl. I saw myself as the decent guy who was teaching her about sex, who was showing her the safe way to use drugs. I was using her, but I didn't want to see it that way.

"Eventually I was aware that something was wrong, that this was not what life should be like, but I didn't know what was causing it, or what to do about it. Several times I stood on a chair in my bedroom, a belt looped around my neck and over the door. I even jumped once, but the belt came loose.

"I started having dreams about being arrested and became increasingly paranoid. I even called the police one night because I thought I saw someone trying to break into my garage. While they were there talking to me, I realized I had been seeing things. And all this time there were several ounces of cocaine in my bedroom. That was the strange thing about my addiction: I felt I was above the law, that I couldn't be caught — but there was some part of me that wanted to get caught, to be done with it. About two years after starting to use cocaine, that wish came true."

One evening Alan made a phone call to a friend, inviting him to a party on the following Saturday. It would be the usual lavish affair — plenty of food, drink, and drugs. Alan had hired ten prostitutes, plus had several x-rated videotapes. What Alan didn't know was that the Federal Drug Enforcement Agency, who had been listening to his phone conversation, was also planning on making it to the party.

At seven o'clock Saturday evening the guests started to arrive. Alan and Hernandez had set out the best china and silver, filled imported decanters with German wines, and had the caterers deliver trays of cheeses, meats, and crackers. On the huge oak dining room table sat twenty silver salt servers filled with cocaine, each with an ornate silver spoon. Everywhere in the house — on end tables, in the bathrooms, beside beds — were mirrors of every size and shape. And at each mirror there was a gold plated razor blade and toot-tube. Alan was ready for the biggest bash of his life.

> "When the bust came, there were 40 people in the house. They started flushing things down the toilets, and throwing things out the windows. Many of the guests had criminal records, and several carried guns. The D.E.A. had received back-up from the F.B.I., the local police, and the county sheriff. There must have been twenty police cars, all with their lights flashing. Nobody resisted at all. I remember saying to the officer who arrested me, 'Thank God, it's all over.'
>
> "I was charged with a series of felonies, including possession of cocaine, possession of criminal tools (the scales for weighing the coke), attempt to carry concealed weapons, possession of Quaaludes, hashish, and other chemicals, and attempted statutory rape (the young girl was at the party). This was only the beginning of the end. The next few months were extremely difficult and several times I didn't manage well at all."

Alan called his father shortly after his arrest. His father told him he was a disgrace to the family and that he never wanted to speak to him. Alan spent a month in a mental institution, where a doctor told him he needed treatment for drug dependency. His lawyer got his trial postponed, and Alan entered a residential chemical dependency treatment center.

The story of his arrest had filled the local newspapers, and his family and friends were constantly being badgered by the press. He had to sell his business and was forced to take a substantial loss. He had to sell his home, cars, and most of his possessions to pay bail, lawyers, etc. His annual income had been about $80,000, so he lost a job capable of providing him with over two and a half million dollars over the next thirty years. The state pulled his insurance license, and his contacts in the business world were gone forever. All his family and friends from his predrug days would have nothing to do with him, and most of his drug friends were in jail or hiding. Alan was pretty much alone in the world, with not much to show for his experience.

> "I thought I was a pretty smart guy. I had read a lot about drugs, had heard about psychological addiction, but I didn't figure I was susceptible. I never wanted to take any addictive drugs and I was very cautious. Even in the '60s, when people started smoking marijuana, I waited a few years before I tried it. I wanted to see if anybody went crazy. I knew I didn't want to do opium, heroin, or anything that was injectable — that would mean I was an addict. I watched people who did coke and they seemed fine, so I figured it was safe. I didn't realize that psychological addiction was at least as powerful, and maybe more powerful than any physical effects.
>
> "The fact that I could afford to buy drugs in large quantities contributed to my problems, but it merely hastened the process along; I got sicker, faster. The last year of my use I spent about $100,000 on drugs. I gave away a lot — to women and other 'friends'— but most

of it I used myself. Some of that money came from savings, some from my business, and some from dealing.

"When I first started dealing, I only sold to a few friends, and only in quantities of an ounce or more. I wanted them to be able to buy good stuff, so I would let them come in at my price. Later on I started cutting the coke, mixing it with other stuff. Sometimes I'd get into a bag I had purchased for someone else. I'd use up some of it and have to cut it a lot when I sold it to them. Eventually my morality with my drug friends dissappeared. I would constantly shortweight them — for every ten grams I sold, I would take out one for myself, and not tell them. I always kept all the rock and crystal for myself — the best part. Toward the end I stopped sharing with others. If they wanted coke, then they could buy some from me. All of this served to alienate me — I became a social recluse. Even when I had big parties, I would often feel isolated from the guests. After my arrest, my sense of isolation became overwhelming.

"After a month of treatment for chemical dependency, I went to a halfway house. While I was there I was served with divorce papers. After six months in the halfway house and five months in therapy, I had to stand trial, was convicted, and was sentenced to serve from three to fifteen years in the state prison.

"My time in jail was very difficult. I knew that I had been wrong and some punishment was in order, but I felt at the time I was being persecuted. The newspapers followed the trial closely, and there was a lot of clamor for a conviction and a stiff penalty. What many people failed to see was that I had already paid a very stiff price; I had virtually nothing left of my life. There were only two things that helped me survive prison without succumbing to the temptations available. One was a sense of stubbornness, even anger. I felt 'they' had taken so much from me already, but they weren't going to take my sobriety. It was all I had left. The other was the new sense of spirituality I had gained from treatment and therapy. While in prison I met a woman from India who told me I could see this as a learning experience. 'Alan,' she said, 'It is as though you have been sent here by God to learn something about yourself, and others.' I tried to see it that way."

Alan served seven months of his sentence, and was released with time off for good behavior. Three and a half years later, he is still on parole and must report regularly to his parole officer. He attends A.A. and N.A. meetings, and is learning to be a chemical dependency counselor.

"I need to be around spiritual people, people who are living my sober lifestyle. I know I'm not ready for the fast-paced business world, but I don't know if I'll ever want to be a part of that. I need to take good care of myself, and I need to be around people I can share my feelings with. I can't allow myself to get emotionally blocked-up or isolated. When the pressure builds up — that's when I want to use drugs again.

"The halfway house I went to was essential for me. I'd spent a lot of years using alcohol and other drugs and I didn't know how to have real feelings. I didn't know how to share myself, how to have female friends I wasn't having sex with, how to have male friends who weren't business competition. I had never had any supportive male friends — guys that I could cry with, that could put their arms around me. I feel both happy and sad thinking about the people I knew at the halfway house. I love them a lot.

"Cocaine literally ate me alive. It is an extremely powerful drug. Users feel that its power is transferred to them, but it's not. I have absolutely no doubt that if I had not been arrested, if my use had not been stopped by intervention, I would be dead today. I would either have succeeded in killing myself, or something else would have happened.

"My life today is difficult. I lost very much. But what I have gained is immeasurable. I am now sober, content, and working towards building a new life. I now have some boundaries in my life. Sometimes I feel a heaviness about my life. When I'd get high, I'd laugh a lot, play jokes on people. Maybe life has become a little more serious to me because I've invested a lot of emotional energy into my recovery. But today my life is much simpler — I don't need two accountants and a lawyer hanging around me.

"After I got out of prison I spent some time in Puerto Rico walking the beach, and there was a guy who would climb the trees and bring down a coconut for fifty cents. It always tasted wonderful — so sweet and quenching. One day, I had no money, and he climbed the tree anyway. When he had sliced it open for me he said, 'God gave me these coconuts. Here, take it. If you have money another day, fine — if not, fine.' I guess I feel that some of the lessons I have learned are like this. If someone else can learn something from the gifts that I have been given, fine."

CONCLUSION

There are certain similarities that are common among chemically dependent people. Richard O. Heilman, M.D., has identified a cluster of eight symptoms of chemical dependency that are often used in diagnosis.[3] Not all chemically dependent people experience all of these symptoms, yet they occur frequently in many people. Several of these symptoms have been represented by the people in the stories just related.

One of the early signs of chemical dependency is **preoccupation with drugs.** Chemically dependent people spend much of their time thinking about past drug experiences, anticipating future use, and devising plans for obtaining drugs.

Katie experienced this symptom by choosing situations where she had easy access to drugs. She worked at the low-paying nightclub because of the availability of chemicals, and eventually abandoned her career plans in the pursuit of drugs. Later, while working as a secretary, she eagerly anticipated the experience of shooting up and could hardly wait for the workday to end. In the end, her entire existence was centered around the process of getting high. Even when she did not have access to drugs, she thought about them and looked forward with excitement and longing for the next opportunity to use them.

As drug use progresses, dependent people often discover they are able to consume larger amounts of drugs. They appear able to function remarkably well after drinking amounts that leave others visibly impaired. **Increased tolerance** to various drugs is a symptom of chemical dependency that is not clearly understood physiologically. However, it often causes dependent people to take increasingly larger doses to achieve the same level of euphoria.

Alan's use of cocaine progressed from an occasional snort to using a gram every few days. He soon found he required a few extra toots to get to the emotional state he was seeking. He slowly began to believe that being high was normal, and that being straight was abnormal. He eventually reached the point of wanting to be in his "normal" condition as much as possible. The time periods between episodes decreased, until at the end he was high on cocaine almost continuously. Usually people who are chemically dependent want to "get high." It becomes the primary reason for using drugs, and the goal is to get to that state as quickly as possible. In alcoholics this is often accomplished by ordering a double martini, a "beer and a bump," etc.

For Katie, this **rapid intake** took the form of only wanting to inject drugs directly. She considered snorting to be too slow and ineffective. Taking pills or drinking alcohol was a last-ditch attempt at euphoria or relief for her.

Sociability becomes less and less important for the chemically dependent. They don't hesitate to use drugs alone, or when others are not taking drugs. At first the pattern of **solitary drug use** may be surreptitious. Dependent people sense a difference in their drug use compared to that of others, and do not wish to draw attention to it. Later, this hiding may break down, and there may be many bouts of solitary drug use.

When Dana was feeling depressed and anti-social, he would confine himself to his room for several days. During these periods he would take drugs continuously, stopping only when he ran out. These binges served to isolate him from his friends and relatives, and his response to this isolation was to use more drugs.

Alan, too, used drugs when he was alone. He would wander around his big house and snort line after line of coke. It made him feel less lonely, he thought, and distracted him from his unhappiness with himself. Later, Alan tooted cocaine alone in his car on the way to business appointments, and in his office before meeting people.

Medicinal use is typical of many people who are dependent on drugs. If they have trouble getting to sleep, they may have a shot of whiskey. If tired, they may take speed or cocaine to give them energy. If they are in physical or emotional pain, they may self-prescribe various chemicals in order to tolerate the discomfort.

Dana used a wide variety of drugs to alter his moods. He enjoyed the effects of LSD, but when he got too jumpy, he would smoke marijuana to calm down. When he needed to attend classes, Dana took speed or snorted coke to "get up" for the occasion.

When Katie was coming down from a coke trip, she would experience emotional turmoil and physical discomfort. To alleviate this she would take tranquilizers or downers to go to sleep. When Katie was up late at night and had to go to work the next day, she took speed, and later cocaine, to give her the "boost" she felt she needed.

Periods of amnesia, or "blackouts," sometimes occur among the chemically dependent. Although more common with those who abuse alcohol or sedatives, blackouts can happen to people who mix different kinds of drugs. When experiencing a blackout, a chemically dependent person cannot remember anything about the time when they are heavily intoxicated.

Katie experienced a very traumatic blackout, remembering nothing past meeting some men in a bar and having a few drinks. She later learned that she had taken several different drugs and gone for a ride in the back of a pick-up truck. She was cut up and badly bruised by bouncing around in the back of the truck, but even after finding out what had really occurred, she still could not remember the events of the evening.

Preoccupation with their supply often affects those who are addicted to drugs, and they tend to maintain close contact with their sources. Alan, Katie, and Dana all turned to dealing drugs, initially for economic reasons, but eventually to help them secure a constant and reliable personal supply. All three also became very guarded about the amount they had, and their generosity with friends fell sharply. "Towards the end I stopped sharing with others," related Alan. "If they wanted coke, then they could buy it from me." For Alan it wasn't the money involved. He needed to protect his supply, to insure that he could always have cocaine whenever he might need it. Alan also carried small amounts of coke with him wherever he went, "just in case."

The final symptom of chemical dependency, as described by Dr. Heilman, relates to **unplanned use of drugs.** Dependent people often establish personal rules about when and how much they will use, and then break those rules. They may decide to have only two drinks at dinner and end up completely intoxicated several hours later.

When Katie and her husband were dealing cocaine, they would take a little bit out to "test it." Their intent was to try a small amount, then sell the remainder, but "all of a sudden it would be two days later and we had shot up $1,000 worth of somebody else's cocaine."

Alan, too, set his own rules of drug use. When he was drinking, he made a point of drinking only on the weekends. Before long, the weekends began at noon on Fridays. Initially he would never have imagined snorting coke while at work; in the end he couldn't imagine not doing it at work.

Dr. Heilman states that someone who has four or more of these eight symptoms on a fairly consistent basis is likely to be chemically dependent. All three of the people whose stories we have just read had most, or all, of these symptoms at one time or another. They were, and are, chemically dependent.

Each of them, however, has learned to live a happy, healthy, and productive life without the need of mood-altering chemicals. Through a process of their own growing awareness and the concern and care of others, they were able to seek out and accept help and guidance. But, because people have different dependency experiences, they can also have individual recovery processes.

Katie's recovery began when she experienced a blackout. It was an event that got her attention, and forced her to look closely at herself. Her fear, coupled with the knowledge of the recent recovery of her ex-husband and another friend, drove her to call a local Alcoholics Anonymous group. She talked with a woman who helped her get through her immediate crisis, and who invited her to attend a meeting that night. Scared to death, Katie went to the meeting. Over the next few days, she and her sponsor worked out a plan for her recovery. Now, after more than a year of sobriety, Katie is going through a chemical dependency counselor training program. She attends A.A. meetings at least once a week, and more often if she feels the need. Her life is starting to work for her, and she is proud of the changes she has been able to make.

Dana knew that things were not right in his life. He suspected that drugs played a part, but it wasn't until he had a serious talk with his sister that he realized how big a part drugs were. Still, he didn't want to believe it. He really felt that his problems were small, and that he could control them. His abstinence lasted only a few days, and after an assessment interview at a chemical dependency treatment center, Dana knew that he could not manage his problems on his own. He stayed at the treatment center for about a month, during which time he learned much about chemical dependency and even more about himself. After treatment, Dana attended weekly A.A. and Narcotics Anonymous meetings. Things appeared to be going well, but after a month he got high. After his binge he knew he would never be able to use drugs again. He lived for a while in a halfway house with other men who had similar problems. Three years later, he is still clean and pleased with the new person that has emerged from within him.

Alan's final recovery began with the intervention of the law. Although he had attended A.A. meetings in years past, Alan felt he had overcome his problem with alcohol, and no longer needed to attend. After his arrest he knew he needed help, but had no idea how to get it until a doctor recognized his symptoms of chemical dependency. After treatment, he lived in a halfway house for drug offenders, and felt that experience was the most valuable for him. He learned much about himself and about healthy human relationships and discovered the strength that people can provide to each other. After the halfway house, Alan entered into some very intensive private therapy sessions. During this therapy, he worked on some personality changes, and solidified his commitment to abstinence. His time spent in prison also aided in his recovery process, even though it was so difficult for him. He knew that if he could survive and maintain his sobriety in prison, then he could face future challenges. After more than three and a half years, Alan is learning to become a chemical dependency counselor. His zest for life and his personal commitment are a model for others, whether chemically dependent or not.

If you, or someone you know, needs advice concerning chemical dependency, it is important to know that help is available. Throughout the United States, and much of the world, there are treatment centers, counseling agencies, and self-help groups such as Alcoholics Anonymous and Narcotics Anonymous. For further information, contact chemical dependency treatment centers, local social service agencies, hospitals or churches.

If someone you know is showing the symptoms of chemical dependency, there are several things that you need to know. Chemical dependency is a progressive disease, and it is fatal if not treated. But the progression of the disease can be stopped and many of the effects can be reversed with appropriate guidance and/or treatment. But whether or not the person you are concerned about seeks help, there are several things that you can do for yourself, which ultimately can benefit both of you.

First, learn all you can about chemical dependency. Read books, attend lectures, and become familiar with the aspects of the disease as it relates to the person you are concerned about. Armed with knowledge, you can be a positive influence.

Second, take care of yourself. Do not accept guilt or blame for the action, or inaction, of the dependent person. Their drug use is not your fault. Attend regular meetings of Al-Anon or Alateen to help you learn to live with a chemically dependent person, whether he or she is recovering or still using. These groups have been very successful in helping chemically dependent people and their families.

Finally, show your concern and love for the chemically dependent person. Encourage him or her to seek appropriate help, and offer support when that person follows through with a recovery plan. By working together, the potentially deadly outcome of the disease of chemical dependency can be stopped.

END NOTES

1. Richard R. Lingeman, *Drugs from A to Z: A Dictionary* (New York: McGraw-Hill, 1974), pp. 45-48.

2. Ernest Jones, *Life and Work of Sigmund Freud, Volume 1 (1856-1900)* (New York: Basic Books, 1953), pp. 82-83. Cited by Edward M. Brecher and the editors of *Consumer Reports,* "Licit and Illicit Drugs" (New York: Consumers Union, 1972), pp. 273-274.

3. Richard O. Heilman, *Early Recognition Of Alcoholism And Other Drug Dependence* (Center City, MN: Hazelden Foundation, 1973), pp. 9-11.